WHAT'S THE 5:2?

A BOOK WITH RECIPES

Carol R. Kotter

Contents

Chapter One

INTRODUCTION

Are there any instances where you tried to lose weight by starving yourself for weeks on end, only to quit because you were fatigued, starved, and just plain cranky about the situation? You're not the only one. Despite the fact that restricting calories is an effective way to lose weight, most individuals give up on diets based on it since they can't keep it up day after day (after day!).

Intermittent fasting is the foundation of the 5:2 Diet. A calorie-restricted phase lasts for two days, after which you can eat normally for the remaining five days of the week. Just two days of consuming a fourth of what you normally consume, sandwiched between days when you aren't fasting, is all it takes. You don't have to deprive yourself of your favourite foods in order to lose weight. Additionally, the 5:2 Diet can lower your chance of developing chronic conditions including heart disease and diabetes..

2 WHAT'S THE 5:2?

To maintain a healthy lifestyle, the 5:2 Diet does not necessitate major lifestyle changes, pricey foods or meal replacements. That's what makes it so great. Fasting may already be a part of your lifestyle without you realising it! At six in the evening, if you don't snack afterward, you'll be fasting for sixteen hours before your first meal of the day, which will be mid-morning. The 5:2 Diet makes fasting a part of your daily routine rather than a side effect of a hectic schedule. There are seventy-seven dishes in this book that may be used on non-fasting days as well, making it an excellent guide for the 5:2 Diet.

The 5:2 Diet is explained in a step-by-step manner in this book to make it easier for you to grasp. You'll be ready to begin your fast when you get to the scrumptious meals in Part Two! Some of the most significant points you'll learn from this book are the following:

a thorough understanding of the 5:2 Diet, its origins, and the principles of fasting

Information on the 5:2 Diet's health advantages and the research behind it is essential.

What to expect in the first month, simple tactics for adjusting to the 5:2 diet, and 10 steps to get you started are all covered in this guide.

Here are some frequently asked questions about the 5:2 Diet and the answers to them.

Information on what to eat and what to avoid on fasting days, as well as low-calorie culinary methods for making all of your meals, are included in this guide.

This book provides meal plans for the first month of your fast, which include many recipes from this book and show exactly how five hundred and six hundred calories look on fasting days.

Advice on how to approach fasting on days when you're not fasting

You'll be able to plan your 5:2 Diet journey with the help of this book. I wish you the best of luck!

Recipes

Salad of spiced shrimp with corn and black beans

• EACH SERVING CONTAINS 354 CALORIES

• TOTAL TIME TO PREPARE: 15 MINUTES

If you're wanting Mexican food, this salad will satisfy your need without the fat and calories. This shrimp dish is spiced with chilli powder and powdered cumin, and brightened with fresh lemon juice.

• SPRAY FOR COOKING

• CHILI POWDER (1 TABLESPOON)

• GARLIC SALT (12 TEASPOON)

12 TEASPOON CUMIN GROUND

• 112 POUNDS PEELED AND DEVEINED MEDIUM SHRIMP

• FRESH LIME JUICE (2 TABLESPOONS)

• 112 CUPS THAWED FROZEN WHOLE-KERNEL CORN

• ¾ CUP SALSA JARRED

• 14 CUP FRESH CILANTRO CHOPPED

• RINSED AND DRAINED ONE 15-OUNCE CAN BLACK BEANS

1. Spray a large nonstick skillet with cooking spray and heat on high.

2. Combine chilli powder, garlic salt, and cumin in a large mixing basin. Toss in the shrimp until they are evenly coated. Place shrimp in pan and cook for 3 minutes, or until pink and cooked through. 1 tablespoon lime juice, stirred into the pan Place the shrimp on a dish. Add corn to the pan and cook for 1 minute. Cook for 1 minute, or until salsa, cilantro, and beans with corn are heated through. 1 tablespoon lime juice is left over. Distribute the beans among four dishes and top with the shrimp.

Chapter Two

Salad with Quinoa, Chicken, Walnuts, and Fruit

SERVES 4

- EACH SERVING CONTAINS 390 CALORIES

- TOTAL TIME TO PREPARE: 40 MINUTES

Quinoa is a high-fiber, high-protein grain that, while bland on its own, pairs nicely with other ingredients to create delectable recipes. Walnuts, which are high in protein, fibre, vitamin E, and omega-3 fatty acids, are also used in this dish.

- SPRAY FOR COOKING

- FOUR BONELESS, SKINLESS CHICKEN BREASTS, 4 OUNCES

- SALT (14 TEASPOON)

- FRESHLY GROUND PEPPER (12 TEASPOON)

- 112 CUPWATER

- QUINOA (34 CUP)

- OLIVE OIL (1 TABLESPOON)

- 3 TABLESPOONS VINEGAR (RED)

- DIJON MUSTARD (1 TEASPOON)

- 1 TABLESPOON ORANGE JUICE (FRESH)

- 1 TEASPOON ZEST OF ORANGE

14 CUP FRESH MINT, CRUMBLED

2 CRUMBLED GREEN ONIONS

- 1 CUP APPLE DICED

- DRIED CHERRIES (12 CUP)

- 2 TABLESPOONS WALNUTS, CRUMBLED

12 CUP RED ONION, DICED

1. Heat a grill pan or a big nonstick skillet over medium-high heat with cooking spray. Season chicken with salt and pepper and cook for 9 minutes, or until no longer pink, flipping once. Remove from the fire and set aside for 2 minutes to cool. Thinly slice into strips.

2. Pour the water into a medium pot and add the quinoa while the chicken cooks. Bring the water to a boil, then reduce to a low heat, cover, and cook for 15 minutes. Refrigerate for 30 minutes after fluffing with a fork.

3. Whisk together the oil, vinegar, mustard, orange juice, orange zest, mint, and green onions in a medium mixing basin. Add the apple, cherries, walnuts, and red onion and mix well. Combine quinoa with it. Serve quinoa on four plates with chicken on top.

Salad with Greek Chicken

SERVES 4

• EACH SERVING CONTAINS 343 CALORIES

• TOTAL TIME TO PREPARE: 25 MINUTES

The simplicity of Greek salad is its beauty. The salad may be served any time of year, but it's especially delicious in the summer, when the key ingredients—tomatoes and cucumbers—are at their freshest. Look for pitted kalamata olives if you want to get the best olives for the dish.

•   CUP VINEGAR OF RED WINE

• OLIVE OIL (2 TABLESPOONS)

• 1 TABLESPOON FRESH DILL, CRUMBLED (OR 1 TEASPOON DRIED)

• GARLIC POWDER (1 TEASPOON)

• SALT (14 TEASPOON)

• FRESHLY GROUND PEPPER (14 TEASPOON)

• 6 CUP ROMAINE LETTUCE, CRUMBLED

• 212 CUPS ROTISSERIE CHICKEN, CHOPPED

2 CRUMBLED MEDIUM TOMATOES

12 CUP RED ONION, FINELY CRUMBLED

• 1 MEDIUM CUCUMBER, PEELED, SEEDED, AND CUT IN HALF

12 CUP BLACK OLIVES, SLICED

12 CUP FETA CHEESE, CRUMBLED

Whisk together the vinegar, oil, dill, garlic powder, salt, and pepper in a large mixing basin. Toss together the lettuce, chicken, tomatoes, onion, cucumber, olives, and feta cheese until completely combined. Serve right away.

Chapter Three

Salad with Skirt Steak and Arugula

SERVES 4

- EACH SERVING CONTAINS 253 CALORIES

- TOTAL TIME TO PREPARE: 25 MINUTES

Arugula, a tasty leafy green with a strong peppery bite, is a good choice for adding a little additional oomph to your salads. The salad pairs perfectly with the grilled skirt steak, dressed in a tangy mustard vinaigrette.

- SKIRT STEAK (1 POUND)

- SALT AND PEPPER, FRESHLY GROUND

- DIJON MUSTARD, 2 TEASPOONS

- 2 TEASPOONS VINEGAR (RED)

- 1 TEASPOON LEMON JUICE (FRESH)

- ½ CUP OIL OF OLIVE

- 2 TABLESPOONS FRESH CILANTRO CHOPPED

- 5 CUPS PACKED ARUGULA

12 RED ONION, SLICED THINLY

- GREEN BEANS, HALVED AND CUT LENGTHWISE, 8 OUNCES

- 1 BUNCH QUARTERED RADISHES

- ONE CUP OF BEANSPROUTS

- 2 CUPS BROCCOLI SLAW (PACKAGED)

3 THINLY SLICED GREEN ONIONS

Preheat the broiler.

2. Season the steak on both sides with salt and pepper. Broil steak for 4 minutes per side on a broiler-safe baking pan, or until desired doneness is reached. Remove from the pan and set aside to cool for 5 minutes before slicing thinly across the grain.

3. Combine mustard, vinegar, lemon juice, oil, cilantro, and a pinch of salt and pepper in a large mixing dish. Toss together the arugula, red onion, green beans, radishes, bean sprouts, broccoli slaw, and green onions. Serve the salad on four plates with the meat on top.

Chapter Four

Smoothie with Chai

SERVES 1

• EACH SERVING CONTAINS 246 CALORIES

• TOTAL TIME TO PREPARE: 40 MINUTES

Black tea, cinnamon, cardamom, black pepper, and other spices are combined in chai tea. It is a popular Indian dish that can now be purchased in most grocery stores.

• ½ CUP WATER IS BOILING

• SUGAR (14 CUP)

• 4 BAGS OF CHAI TEA

• 2 CUPS ICE

• 12% MILK (12 CUP)

1. Combine boiling water, sugar, and chai tea bags in a small bowl. Steep for 5 minutes, covered. Remove the tea bags and chill the tea for 30 minutes or until completely cold.

2. In a blender, combine the tea, ice, and milk and blend until smooth. Serve right away.

Chapter Five

Yogurt Citrus Parfait

SERVES 4

- EACH SERVING CONTAINS 180 CALORIES

- TOTAL TIME TO PREPARE: 5 MINUTES

Greek yoghurt is high in protein and makes a delicious snack. To avoid the added sugars found in some yoghurts, choose the plain version and flavour it yourself. Choose something sweet, something fruity, and something crunchy as a general rule. Honey, clementines, and pistachios are used in this dish.

- 3 CUPS NONFAT PLAIN GREEK YOGURT

- VANILLA EXTRACT (1 TEASPOON)

- 4 HONEY TEASPOONS

- 28 SECTIONS OF CLEMENTINE

- 14 CUP UNSALTED DRY-ROASTED CHOPED PISTACHIOS

14   WHAT'S THE 5:2?

1. Combine yoghurt and vanilla extract in a medium mixing basin. Fill 4 parfait glasses with 13 cup yoghurt each. 12 teaspoon honey, 5 clementine segments, and 12 tablespoon pistachios are sprinkled on top.

2. Add a quarter of the remaining yoghurt, 12 teaspoon honey, 2 clementine segments, and 12 tablespoon pistachios to each parfait.

Chapter Six

Crispy Cinnamon-Sugar

SERVES 4

• EACH SERVING CONTAINS 89 CALORIES

• TOTAL TIME TO PREPARE: 20 MINUTES

Despite the lack of oil or butter, these chips are surprisingly crisp and tasty. As they bake, keep an eye on them since they can easily burn around the edges.

• 1 SUGAR TABLESPOON

• 14 TEASPOON CINNAMON, GROUND

• TWO FLOUR TORTILLAS, 8 INCHES

• 1 WATER TABLESPOON

Preheat the oven to 350 degrees Fahrenheit.

2. Combine sugar and cinnamon in a small bowl. Brush both sides of the tortillas lightly with water and then sprinkle with the cinnamon-sugar mixture. Cut each tortilla into 12 wedges and place on a cookie sheet in a single layer. Bake for 15 minutes or until golden brown. Before serving, chill the cookies on a wire rack.

Chapter Seven

Chips of Plantain

SERVES 4

- EACH SERVING CONTAINS 190 CALORIES

- TOTAL TIME TO PREPARE: 9 MINUTES

Plantains resemble gigantic bananas, but they must be cooked before consumption. They can also be difficult to peel, so use a sharp knife and proceed with caution. They are high in vitamins A and C as well as other minerals.

- OLIVE OIL (1 TABLESPOON)

- PEELED AND CUT INTO 14-INCH DIAGONAL SLICES 2 PLANTAINS

- SALT (14 TEASPOON)

- GROUND RED PEPPER, 18 TEASPOON

Heat the oil in a large nonstick skillet over medium heat. Cook for 3 minutes on each side, or until plantain slices are golden and crispy. Before serving, remove from the pan and season with salt and pepper.

Chapter Eight

Dried Fruit and Nuts Glazed

SERVES 4

- EACH SERVING CONTAINS 388 CALORIES

- TOTAL TIME TO PREPARE: 15 MINUTES

Consider it a spicier version of trail mix. It's fully adjustable based on your preferences, so use any nuts, seeds, and dried fruit you want. To save time, buy the nuts already chopped.

- SPRAY FOR COOKING

- 1 TEASPOON BUTTER (UNSALTED)

- HONEY (14 CUP)

- SLIVERED ALMONDS (1/4 CUP)

14 CUP HAZELNUTS, CRUMBLED

- 14 CUP CRUMBLED PECANS

- SUNFLOWER SEEDS (14 CUP)

12 TEASPOON CINNAMON, GROUND

- SALT (14 TEASPOON)

- 14 TEASPOON CARDAMOM GROUND

- GROUND CLOVES DASH

RAISINS (1 CUP)

1. Use parchment paper or foil to line a baking pan. Set it aside after spraying it with cooking spray.

2. Melt butter in a large nonstick skillet over medium-high heat. Cook for 2 minutes, or until the honey begins to bubble around the edges. Combine the almonds, hazelnuts, pecans, sunflower seeds, cinnamon, salt, cardamom, and cloves in a mixing bowl. Cook, stirring regularly, for 8 minutes or until the nuts turn brown. Place raisins on a baking pan and let aside to cool completely before serving.

Chapter Nine

Roasted Nuts, Sweet and Spicy

SERVES 4

• EACH SERVING CONTAINS 180 CALORIES

• TOTAL TIME TO PREPARE: 23 MINUTES

Roasted nuts are nothing new, but they are enhanced by the addition of Indian spices such as cardamom and cloves. Nuts are a terrific snack since they're high in protein and unsaturated fat, which will keep you full until your next meal. Do you prefer things a little spicier? Toss in some freshly ground red pepper.

• 112 TEASPOONS BROWN SUGAR PACKED

• 112 HONEY TEASPOONS

• CANOLA OIL (1 TEASPOON)

• 34 TEASPOON CINNAMON, GROUND

- SALT, 18 TEASPOON

- 1 TEASPOON CARDAMOM GROUND

- GROUND CLOVES TEASPOON

- A SPRINKLE OF FRESHLY GROUND PEPPER

14 CUP ALMONDS, BLANCHED

- CASHEWS (14 CUP)

HAZELNUTS (1/4 CUP)

Preheat the oven to 350 degrees Fahrenheit.

2. Combine brown sugar, honey, oil, cinnamon, salt, cardamom, cloves, and pepper in a medium microwave-safe bowl. Stir after 30 seconds in the microwave. Toss the nuts in the sugar mixture to coat them.

3. Spread nuts equally on a baking sheet lined with parchment paper. Preheat oven to 350°F and bake for 15 minutes, or until golden brown. Cool completely before serving.

4 SERVINGS • 260 CALORIES PER SERVING PEANUT BUTTER OATMEAL BALLS

- TOTAL TIME TO PREPARE: 25 MINUTES

These stimulating nibbles are packed with fibre, protein, and healthy fat to keep you full. If you don't like peanuts, you can roll them in any other crushed nut. These are delicious at room temperature or straight from the fridge.

- OLD-FASHIONED ROLLED OATS (14 CUP)

- 1 TABLESPOON ALMONDS, CRUMBLED

- 1 TABLESPOON FLAXSEED, GROUND

- CHIA SEEDS 112 TEASPOONS

- A BIT OF CINNAMON

- A BIT OF SALT

- CREAMY PEANUT BUTTER (112) TABLESPOONS

HONEY, 1 TABLESPOON

- VANILLA EXTRACT DASH

- MINI CHOCOLATE CHIPS (1 TABLESPOON)

- 12 CUP CRUSHED PEANUTS FOR BALL COATING

1. Combine oats, almonds, flaxseed, chia seeds, cinnamon, and salt in a large mixing dish.

2. Melt the peanut butter in a microwave-safe bowl for 20 to 30 seconds, or until completely melted; set aside to cool slightly. Pour peanut butter mixture over oats after adding honey and vanilla. Fold in chocolate chips once the batter is well mixed and sticking together.

3. Form dough into four balls with your hands, then roll them in crushed peanuts.

Chapter Ten

Banana and Peanut Butter Roll-Ups

SERVES 4

• EACH SERVING CONTAINS 367 CALORIES

• TOTAL TIME TO PREPARE: 8 MINUTES

The winning mix of peanut butter and bananas is folded up in a whole-wheat tortilla to provide a convenient chevalier chevalier chevalier chevalier chevalier chevalier chevalier chevalier chevalier chevalier cheval If you don't have wheat germ, you may leave it out, but it provides crunch, protein, and fibre.

• 12 CUP LOW-FAT PEANUT BUTTER

• 13 CUP LOW-FAT VANILLA YOGURT

• 2 SLICED BANANAS

• ORANGE JUICE (1 TABLESPOON)

• FOUR FAT-FREE WHOLE-WHEAT TORTILLAS, 8 INCHES

• 2 TABLESPOONS WHEAT GERM WITH HONEY-CRUNCH

• 14 TEASPOON CINNAMON, GROUND

1. Combine peanut butter and yoghurt in a small bowl and whisk until smooth. Toss the bananas with the orange juice in a separate small bowl.

2. Spread 3 tablespoons peanut butter mixture over each tortilla, leaving 12 inch around the borders naked. Place roughly 13 cup banana slices on top in a single layer.

3. Combine wheat germ and cinnamon in a small basin. Sprinkle the banana slices on top, roll them up, then cut each one into six pieces.

Chapter Eleven

Sandwiches with pear, peanut butter, and cream cheese

SERVES 4

• EACH SERVING CONTAINS 355 CALORIES

• TOTAL TIME TO PREPARE: 12 MINUTES

Carbohydrates, fat, and protein are all important components of a healthy snack. This one covers all of those bases and then some. If an Anjou pear is unavailable, use an Asian pear or apple instead.

14 CUP SOFTENED CREAM CHEESE

• MAPLE SYRUP (1 TABLESPOON)

• 14 TEASPOON CINNAMON, GROUND

• A BIT OF SALT

• TOASTED CINNAMON-RAISIN BREAD, 4 SLICES

• CRUNCHY PEANUT BUTTER (12 CUP)

• THINLY SLICED ANJOU PEAR

1. Combine cream cheese, maple syrup, cinnamon, and salt in a medium mixing bowl.

2. Spread 2 teaspoons peanut butter and 1 tablespoon cream cheese mixture on each slice of bread. Serve with pear slices on top.

Figs stuffed with blue cheese and prosciutto

SERVES 4

• EACH SERVING CONTAINS 263 CALORIES

• TOTAL TIME TO PREPARE: 12 MINUTES

Although these might be eaten raw, the tastes are enhanced when the figs are cooked. Make sure the grill is set on medium-high to crisp the prosciutto and melt the blue cheese softly.

CUT 12 CUP BLUE CHEESE INTO 16 CUBES

• 8 HALVED BLACK MISSION FIGURES

• 8 PROSCIUTTO SLICES, HALVED LENGTHWISE

• OLIVE OIL (2 TABLESPOONS)

• SALT AND PEPPER, FRESHLY GROUND

1. Heat the grill to medium-high. On each fig half, place a bit of blue cheese. Wrap a strip of prosciutto around each fig half, making sure to overlap the ends and cover the cheese.

2. Grill figs for 2 minutes on each side, or until prosciutto begins to crisp. Before serving, spray warm figs with oil and season with salt and pepper.

Chapter Thirteen

Popcorn with Cheesy Garlic

SERVES 3

• EACH SERVING CONTAINS 250 CALORIES

• TOTAL TIME TO PREPARE: 5 MINUTES

Popcorn is a nutritious food that comes in a variety of tastes. Place kernels in a glass dish and microwave for 4 to 5 minutes, or until popping slows, if you don't have an air popper.

• 1 TABLESPOON BUTTER (UNSALTED)

• OLIVE OIL (1 TABLESPOON)

• 1 PRESSED GARLIC CLOVE

• DRIED THYME (12 TEASPOON)

• DRIED BASIL (14 TEASPOON)

• 8 CUP POPCORN, PLAIN POPPED

• 34 CUP PARMESAN CHEESE, GRATED

1. Melt the butter, oil, and garlic in a small saucepan over medium-low heat. Cook for 1 to 2 minutes, stirring regularly, or until garlic is tender. Stir in the thyme and basil.

2. Place popcorn in a large mixing bowl and sprinkle with butter mixture, swirling constantly. Toss in the cheese once the popcorn is evenly coated.

Chapter Fourteen

Nuggets of Mozzarella Crunch

SERVES 4

• EACH SERVING CONTAINS 91 CALORIES

• TOTAL TIME TO PREPARE: 10 MINUTES

Although everyone enjoys mozzarella sticks, the deep-fried snack is not a healthy option. This recipe asks for baking instead of frying and uses premade string cheese.

•   CUP CRUMBS OF PANKO BREAD

• EGG SUBSTITUTE: 3 TABLESPOONS

• THREE PART-SKIM MOZZARELLA STRING-CHEESE STICKS (1 OUNCE)

• SPRAY FOR COOKING

• 14 CUP MARINARA SAUCE WITH LOWER SODIUM FOR DIPPING

Preheat the oven to 425 degrees Fahrenheit.

2. Toast the bread crumbs in a medium skillet over medium heat for 2 minutes, turning constantly. In a shallow bowl, place bread crumbs. Fill another shallow dish with the egg substitute.

3. Cut mozzarella sticks into 1-inch pieces with a sharp knife. Dip each piece of cheese in the egg substitute and then in the bread crumbs, one at a time.

4. Spray a baking sheet with cooking spray and lay out the cheese. 3 minutes in the oven, or until cheese is softened and warmed through

5. Cook for 1 minute in the microwave, stirring halfway through. With the dipping sauce, serve the mozzarella slices.

Chapter Fifteen

Poppers de Jalapeo

SERVES 4

• EACH SERVING CONTAINS 255 CALORIES

• TOTAL TIME TO PREPARE: 15 MINUTES

When deep fried, jalapeo poppers are a terrific appetiser or snack, but they can be heavy in fat and calories. To lighten the burden, these are baked. When sowing the jalapeos, make sure to remove the ribs as well, as they can also transport heat.

• 4 OUNCES SOFTENED CREAM CHEESE

12 CUP SHARP CHEDDAR CHEESE, GRATED

• SALT AND PEPPER, FRESHLY GROUND

• 6 HALVED, SEEDED, AND DERIBBED JALAPEOS

1. Preheat oven to 450 degrees Fahrenheit.

2. Combine cream cheese and cheddar cheese in a small mixing dish. Salt & pepper to taste. Fill each half of a jalapeo with about 1 spoonful of the cheese mixture.

3. Place the filled peppers on a baking sheet lined with parchment paper. Bake for 10 minutes, flipping sheet halfway through, or until cheese is golden and bubbling. Allow to cool before serving.

Chapter Sixteen

Nachos with the Works

SERVES 4

• EACH SERVING CONTAINS 412 CALORIES

• TOTAL TIME TO PREPARE: 30 MINUTES

By heaping toppings onto each chip rather than piling them on top of one another, you can ensure that every bite contains all of the tastes. The use of baked tortilla chips reduces fat, and with all the toppings, you won't notice.

• LEAN GROUND BEEF, 8 OUNCES

12 CUP JARRED ROASTED RED BELL PEPPERS, CHOPPED

• CHILI POWDER (1 TEASPOON)

• DRIED OREGANO (12 TEASPOON)

• SALT (14 TEASPOON)

- ONE 14.5-OUNCE CAN UNDRAINED TOMATOES WITHOUT SALT

1 CRUSHED GARLIC CLOVE

- SPRAY FOR COOKING

- ONE FAT-FREE REFRIED BEANS WITH MILD CHILES (16-OUNCE CAN)

- DIVIDE 14 CUP MINCED FRESH CILANTRO

14 CUP GREEN ONIONS, CRUMBLED, DIVIDED

- 26 TORTILLA CHIPS (BAKED)

- 1 CUP MONTEREY JACK CHEESE, SHREDDED

- 3 TABLESPOONS SOUR CREAM (LOW-FAT)

Preheat the oven to 375 degrees Fahrenheit.

2. Brown the beef in a large nonstick skillet over medium-high heat, turning to break it up, for 10 minutes. Bell peppers, chilli powder, oregano, salt, tomatoes, and garlic are added to the pan. Cook, stirring occasionally, for 8 minutes or until thick.

3. Heat a second skillet covered with cooking spray over medium heat. 2 tablespoons cilantro, 2 tablespoons green onions, beans Cook for 2 minutes, or until thoroughly heated. Arrange the chips in a single layer on a baking sheet. Top each

chip with the warm bean mixture with meat and cheese. Bake for 9 minutes, or until the cheese is completely melted.

4. Serve immediately with sour cream, remaining cilantro, and remaining green onions.

Chapter Seventeen

Chicken Wings Without Bones

SERVES 4

• EACH SERVING CONTAINS 493 CALORIES

• TOTAL TIME TO PREPARE: 40 MINUTES

Pan-frying the chicken tenders gives them a beautiful crispy texture without using as much oil as deep-frying. This vinegar-based variant is far lighter than buffalo sauce, which is virtually entirely butter. Are you unsure which hot sauce to use? Frank's RedHot is an excellent option.

• 2/3 CUP LOW-FAT SOUR CREAM

• CRUMBLED BLUE CHEESE (12 CUP)

• WHITE VINEGAR, 4 TABLESPOONS

• DIVIDED 34 TEASPOON CAYENNE PEPPER

• 3 TABLESPOONS BUTTERMILK WITHOUT FAT

- 3 TABLESPOONS SAUCE (HOT)

- CHICKEN TENDERS, 2 POUNDS

- WHOLE-WHEAT FLOUR, 6 TABLESPOONS

CORNMEAL, 6 TABLESPOONS

- CANOLA OIL (2 TABLESPOONS)

CARROT STICKS, 2 CUP

- CELERY STICKS, 2 CUP

1. Combine sour cream, blue cheese, 1 tablespoon vinegar, and 14 tsp cayenne pepper in a small bowl. Refrigerate covered.

2. Combine buttermilk, 2 tablespoons hot sauce, and 2 tablespoons vinegar in a large mixing basin. Toss in the chicken to coat. Allow 10 minutes for flavours to meld before serving.

3. Combine flour and cornmeal in a shallow dish.

4. Combine the remaining 1 tablespoon spicy sauce and 1 tablespoon vinegar in a small bowl.

5. Remove chicken from marinade and cover evenly with flour mixture. 12 teaspoon cayenne pepper, on both sides of the chicken

6. Heat 1 tablespoon oil in a large nonstick skillet over medium heat. Add half of the chicken pieces and heat for 3 to 4 minutes per side, or until golden brown and cooked through. Replace the chicken and the remaining 1 tablespoon of oil. Drizzle remaining hot sauce mixture over chicken and serve with sour cream dip, carrots, and celery.

94 CALORIES PER SERVING • Parmesan-Crusted Portobello Caps

• TOTAL TIME TO PREPARE: 20 MINUTES

Dieters will like sharp, firm cheese. Even a dab of it provides dishes a taste boost without adding too many calories. This dish blends savoury Parmesan and meaty mushrooms for a filling low-calorie supper.

• 2 TABLESPOONS PARMESAN CHEESE, FRESHLY GRATED

• 1 TABLESPOON FRESH BASIL, MINCED (OR 1 TEASPOON DRIED)

• 1 LIGHTLY BEATEN EGG

• 1 WHITE EGG, LIGHTLY BEATEN

• 4 CAPS OF PORTOBELLO MUSHROOMS

• 2 TABLESPOONS FLOUR (ALL-PURPOSE)

• OLIVE OIL (1 TABLESPOON)

• FRESH LEMON JUICE (2 TABLESPOONS)

Preheat the oven to 400 degrees Fahrenheit.

2. Combine Parmesan, basil, egg, and egg white in a small mixing dish.

3. Gently mix mushrooms in flour in a sealable plastic bag until evenly coated.

4. Heat oil in a large nonstick skillet over medium heat. In an egg mixture, coat the mushrooms. In a skillet, cook mushrooms for 2 minutes on each side, or until light brown. Pour lemon juice over the mushrooms. Remove pan from heat.

5. Bake mushrooms for 10 minutes or until tender in a baking dish. Allow to cool before serving.

Chapter Eighteen

Sandwich with Tomato and Grilled Cheese

SERVES 1

• EACH SERVING CONTAINS 300 CALORIES

• TOTAL TIME TO PREPARE: 10 MINUTES

This sandwich, inspired by the classic combination of grilled cheese and tomato soup, will satisfy your comfort food desires. Instead of using butter to pan-fry the sandwich, this recipe uses heart-healthy canola oil, which is low in saturated fat.

• 2 WHOLE-WHEAT BREAD SLICES

• CANOLA OIL (1 TABLESPOON)

• REDUCED-FAT PROVOLONE CHEESE, 1 SLICE (APPROXIMATELY 1 OUNCE)

1 TEASPOON WHOLE-GRAIN MAYONNAISE

• BABY SPINACH (14 CUP)

1 THINLY SLICED TOMATO

1. Brush one side of each piece of bread with oil using a pastry brush. Top one slice with cheese, mustard, spinach, and tomato, oiled side down. Place the remaining slice of bread on top, oiled side up.

2. For about 3 minutes, heat a cast-iron or heavy skillet over medium heat. Transfer the sandwich to the pan with a spatula. Cook for 1 minute, pushing the sandwich into the skillet with the spatula to brown the bottom. Repeat with the other side of the sandwich; the cheese should have melted. Serve by halves the sandwich.

Chapter Nineteen

Quesadillas with black beans and cheese

SERVES 4

- EACH SERVING CONTAINS 377 CALORIES

- TOTAL TIME TO PREPARE: 15 MINUTES

If you're missing taco night because of your new healthy lifestyle, make your own fiesta with these fiber- and protein-rich quesadillas. The best aspect about this recipe is that it can be prepared in a flash for four people, giving quick lunch a whole new meaning.

- DRAINED AND RINSED ONE 15-OUNCE CAN BLACK BEANS

12 CUP MONTEREY JACK CHEESE, SHREDDED

12 CUP FRESHLY MADE SALSA

- FOUR WHOLE-WHEAT TORTILLAS, 8 INCHES

- CANOLA OIL, 2 TEASPOONS

• 1 DICED AVOCADO

1. Combine the beans, cheese, and 14 cup salsa in a medium mixing basin. Lay each tortilla down and spread 12 cup of bean mixture on half of each. Fold the tortillas over and carefully press them together.

2. Heat 1 teaspoon oil in a large nonstick skillet over medium heat. Cook two quesadillas at a time until golden brown, about 2 minutes per side. Turn off the heat. Continue with the remaining quesadillas.

3. To serve, add the remaining 14 cup salsa and avocado to the quesadillas.

Chapter Twenty

Tostadas with cheese and roasted vegetables and beans

SERVES 4

• EACH SERVING CONTAINS 463 CALORIES

• TOTAL TIME TO PREPARE: 50 MINUTES

Roasting vegetables is a terrific technique to get the most flavour out of them while spending the least amount of time cooking them. Any leftover vegetables from this dish can be combined into a scramble or incorporated into an omelette the next day.

BUTTON MUSHROOMS, 10 OUNCES, TRIMMED AND QUARTERED

• 2 ZUCCHINI, LENGTHWISELY SLICED

• 2 SEEDED AND CUT INTO 112-INCH PIECES RED BELL PEPPERS

- OLIVE OIL (3 TABLESPOONS)

- SALT

- 8 CORN TORTILLAS, SMALL

- ONE 15-OUNCE REFRIED BEANS CANNON

- 4 OUNCES (ABOUT 1 CUP) CHEDDAR CHEESE, GRATED

- 4 TABLESPOONS SOUR CREAM (LOW-FAT) (OPTIONAL)

- CILANTRO LEAVES, FRESH (OPTIONAL)

- HEATED SAUCE (OPTIONAL)

1. Preheat oven to 450 degrees Fahrenheit.

2. Line two baking sheets with mushrooms, zucchini, and bell peppers. Season each batch with salt and 1 tablespoon of oil. Roast vegetables for 20 to 25 minutes, until soft, stirring halfway through and switching baking sheets. Remove the vegetables from the oven and place them in a medium mixing dish.

3. Arrange the tortillas on the same baking sheets and brush one side of each with the remaining tablespoon of oil. Fill the tortillas with refried beans and cheese. Bake for 5 to 7 minutes, or until cheese has melted and beans are heated. Fill each tortilla with the vegetables and a dollop of sour cream, a sprinkling of cilantro, and a splash of spicy sauce, if desired.

Chapter Twenty-one

Risotto with Butternut Squash and Barley

SERVES 4

- EACH SERVING CONTAINS 427 CALORIES

- TOTAL TIME TO PREPARE: 50 MINUTES

When it comes to calorie restriction, eating more whole grains is a good idea because they suppress your appetite by keeping you feeling full for longer. Barley, which is used in place of conventional risotto in this recipe, decreases blood cholesterol, helps control blood sugar levels, and aids digestion.

- OLIVE OIL (2 TABLESPOONS)

- 1 BUTTERNUT SQUASH, PEELED, SEEDED, AND CUT INTO 1-INCH PIECES (ABOUT 112 POUNDS)

1 FINELY CRUMBLED ONION

- DIVIDED 34 TEASPOON SALT

- DIVIDEd 14 TEASPOON FRESHLY GROUND PEPPER

- 1 CUP BARLEY PEARL

- ½ CUP WHITE WINE, DRY

- 3 CUPS VEGETABLE BROTH WITH LOW SODIUM

- 1 CUP BABY SPINACH IN PACKAGE

- 12 CUP (APPROXIMATELY 2 OUNCES) GRATED FRESH PARMESAN

- 1 TABLESPOON BUTTER (UNSALTED)

Preheat the oven to 400 degrees Fahrenheit.

2. Heat the oil in a Dutch oven or a heavy oven-safe pot over medium heat. 5 minutes, stirring frequently, until squash, onion, salt, and pepper soften. Cook for 1 minute after adding the barley. Pour in the wine and simmer, stirring frequently, for 1 minute, or until the liquid has evaporated. Bring the broth to a boil, then cover and place the saucepan in the oven. Preheat oven to 350°F and bake for 35–40 minutes, or until barley is soft.

3. Turn off the oven. Serve immediately with spinach, Parmesan, and butter.

Chapter Twenty-two

Lasagna with Ricotta and Eggplant

SERVES 4

• EACH SERVING CONTAINS 378 CALORIES

• TOTAL TIME TO PREPARE: 30 MINUTES

Eggplant Parmesan may be a thing of the past for you, but this delicious baked dish could help you overcome a yearning. For carb-conscious dieters and reluctant veggie eaters, this no-noodle meal is a fantastic choice.

• 12 POUND HALVED AND SEEDED PLUM TOMATOES

1 CLOVE OF GARLIC

• OLIVE OIL, 4 TABLESPOONS

• DIVIDE 1 TEASPOON SALT

• DIVIDEd 34 TEASPOON FRESHLY GROUND PEPPER

- 2 EGGPLANTS (EACH ABOUT 112 POUNDS), CUT INTO 14-INCH SLICES LENGTHWISE

- 1 RICOTTA CUP

- 1 EGG

12 CUP FRESH BASIL, CRUMBLED

- 14 CUP PARMESAN OR ASIAGO CHEESE, FRESHLY GRATED

- 4 CUPS GREENS MIXED

Preheat the broiler.

2. Pulse tomatoes, garlic, 1 tablespoon oil, 14 teaspoon salt, and 14 teaspoon pepper in a food processor or blender.

3. Using a pastry brush, evenly cover the eggplant slices with 2 tablespoons of oil. 12 teaspoon salt and 14 teaspoon pepper on each side Place eggplant slices in a single layer on a broiler-safe baking sheet and broil 3 to 4 minutes on each side, until tender and browned.

4. Preheat the oven to 400°F.

5. In a small mixing bowl, combine ricotta, egg, basil, the remaining 14 teaspoon salt, and the remaining 14 teaspoon pepper.

6. Pour half of the tomato sauce into an 8-inch square baking dish and distribute evenly. One-third of the eggplant slices

should be used to make a single layer. Half of the ricotta mixture should be spread on top of the eggplant layer. One-third of the eggplant slices should be used to make a single layer of eggplant. On top of this layer, spread the remaining ricotta. Finish with a final eggplant layer. Spread the Parmesan cheese evenly over the top layer.

7. Bake for 15 to 20 minutes, or until the lasagna is bubbling. Before serving, remove from the heat and set aside for 10 minutes.

8. Arrange mixed greens on individual plates. Season with salt and pepper and drizzle with the remaining 1 tablespoon oil. Serve with the lasagna.

4 SERVINGS Whole-Wheat Spaghetti Carbonara • 385 CALORIES PER SERVING • TOTAL PREP TIME: 30 MINUTES

You may be watching what you eat, but you can indulge in the delicious things in moderation. This dish includes bacon, demonstrating that a little goes a long way in terms of flavour. If you only have standard pasta on hand, go ahead and use it; but, the whole-wheat version provides over 10 grammes of fibre per serving.

• WHOLE-WHEAT SPAGHETTI (8 OUNCES)

• 2 CUPS THAWED FROZEN PEAS

3 MINCED GARLIC CLOVES

• 4 BACON STRIPS (THICK CUT)

• ROOM TEMPERATURE 2 EGGS

• DIVIDE 34 CUP FINELY SHREDDED PARMESAN CHEESE

• SALT (14 TEASPOON)

• FRESHLY GROUND PEPPER (14 TEASPOON)

1. Bring water to a boil in a big saucepan. Cook for about 8 minutes, or until the spaghetti is cooked (refer to package directions for accurate cooking time). Stir in peas and garlic after 5 minutes of simmering.

2. While the pasta is cooking, fry the bacon in a nonstick skillet over medium heat. To absorb the fat, place the bacon on a platter lined with paper towels. Whisk together the saved bacon drippings, eggs, 12 cup Parmesan, salt, and pepper in a large mixing basin. Chop the bacon and add it to the egg mixture.

3. When the pasta and peas are done, drain the cooking water and save aside 34 cup. Quickly incorporate the pasta, peas, and water with the egg mixture. Allow 5 minutes for the sauce to thicken, stirring regularly. Before serving, divide the spaghetti among four bowls and top with the remaining 14 cup Parmesan.

Chapter Twenty-three

Shrimp with Lemon-Garlic

SERVES 4

• EACH SERVING CONTAINS 117 CALORIES

• TOTAL TIME TO PREPARE: 16 MINUTES

When it comes to seasoning a meal, the fragrant combination of lemon and garlic can't be beat. When you add butter to the mix, as this recipe does, you've got yourself a winner. If you can't find lemon-pepper spice, a squeeze of fresh lemon can be used to finish the shrimp.

• SPRAY FOR COOKING

• LARGE SHRIMP, PEELED AND DEVEINED, 114 POUNDS

• ¼ CUP LEMON JUICE, FRESH

• 2 TABLESPOONS MELTED UNSALTED BUTTER

3 MINCED GARLIC CLOVES

WORCESTERSHIRE SAUCE, 1 TEASPOON

- 34 TEASPOON LEMON-PEPPER SAUCE

- 14 TEASPOON RED PEPPER, GROUND

- 2 TABLESPOONS FRESH PARSLEY, CRUMBLED

Preheat the oven to 425 degrees Fahrenheit.

2. Using cooking spray, coat a 9-by-13-inch baking dish. Arrange the shrimp in a single layer in the dish.

3. Combine the lemon juice, butter, garlic, Worcestershire sauce, lemon-pepper spice, and red pepper in a small mixing bowl. Pour the sauce over the shrimp.

4. Bake shrimp for 9 minutes, or until cooked through and pink. Remove from heat and top with parsley before serving.

Chapter Twenty-four

Ceviche with shrimp and jalapeo

SERVES 4

• EACH SERVING CONTAINS 80 CALORIES

• TOTAL TIME TO PREPARE: 35 MINUTES

This chilled meal is a balanced blend of huge tastes and very little calories, tantalising the palette with a combination of citrus and spice. If you can't get jicama, use julienned radishes instead, but keep in mind that the latter are more peppery.

• COOKED 12 POUND PEELED LARGE SHRIMP

• FRESH LIME JUICE (2 TABLESPOONS)

• 2 TABLESPOONS FRESH CILANTRO CHOPPED

1 GREEN ONION, CHOPPED 12 GARLIC CLOVES, MINCED

12 SEEDED, DERIBBED, AND DICED RED BELL PEPPER

- 12 CUP PEELED AND CUT JICAMA

- SECTIONS OF 14 CUP ORANGE

- 12 SEEDED, DERIBBED, AND MINCED JALAPEOS

- A BIT OF SALT

Combine all ingredients in a large mixing bowl. Allow at least 30 minutes for chilling. Cool before serving.

Chapter Twenty-five

Baked Spicy Tilapia

SERVES 4

- EACH SERVING CONTAINS 230 CALORIES

- TOTAL TIME TO PREPARE: 14 MINUTES

Cooking for health does not have to be boring. To add flavour to your foods while keeping calorie counts low, reach for your spice rack. This recipe's chilli spice blend amps up the mild, delicate tilapia for a more thrilling lunch.

- CHILI POWDER (1 TEASPOON)

- CAYENNE PEPPER (14 TEASPOON)

- GARLIC POWDER (1 TEASPOON)

- SALT (1 TEASPOON)

- FRESHLY GROUND PEPPER (12 TEASPOON)

• 4 TILAPIA FILLETS, 6 OUNCES

• OLIVE OIL (2 TABLESPOONS)

• WEDGES OF LIME (OPTIONAL)

1. Preheat oven to 450 degrees Fahrenheit.

2. Combine chilli powder, cayenne pepper, garlic powder, salt, and pepper in a small mixing dish. Distribute the spice mixture equally across both sides of the tilapia fillets.

3. Brush 1 tablespoon of oil onto a baking sheet. Arrange the fish in a single layer on the baking sheet. 1 tablespoon oil remains to be drizzled over the fish. Bake for 8 minutes, or until flaky and golden brown. With lime wedges on the side (if using).

Chapter Twenty-six

Spaghetti with Lemon-Caper Salmon

SERVES 4

- EACH SERVING CONTAINS 462 CALORIES

- TOTAL TIME TO PREPARE: 20 MINUTES

This dish helps you put up a near-perfect meal in under 20 minutes, thanks to whole-grain pasta, lean protein, and spinach on the side. Lemon zest is called for in the recipe, and it's worth it for the vivid burst of strong citrus flavour it adds to the platter.

- SPAGHETTI (12 POUNDS WHOLE-WHEAT)

1 MINCED GARLIC CLOVE

- OLIVE OIL (3 TABLESPOONS)

- SALT (12 TEASPOON)

- FRESHLY GROUND PEPPER (12 TEASPOON)

14 CUP FRESH BASIL LEAVES, CRUMBLED

CAPERS (3 TABLESPOONS)

• ONE LEMON ZEST

• FRESH LEMON JUICE (2 TABLESPOONS)

• FOUR FILLETS OF SALMON, 4 OUNCES

• 2 CUP BABY SPINACH, PACKED

1. Bring salted water to a boil in a large stockpot or saucepan over high heat. Cook for about 8 minutes, or until the spaghetti is al dente (refer to package directions for accurate cooking time). Drain the pasta and place it in a big mixing bowl. Mix in the garlic, 2 tablespoons oil, salt, and pepper until smooth. Combine basil, capers, lemon zest, and lemon juice in a mixing bowl.

2. Heat the remaining tablespoon of oil in a large nonstick skillet over medium-high heat. Cook the salmon for 2 minutes on each side, until medium rare. Place fish in a serving dish.

3. Divide the spinach evenly among the serving bowls. Finish with a slice of salmon and a quarter of the spaghetti mixture.

Chapter Twenty-seven

Salmon with Spinach and Pepper Sauté in Honey-Soy Sauce

SERVES 4

• EACH SERVING CONTAINS 321 CALORIES

• TOTAL TIME TO PREPARE: 20 MINUTES

If you want to create a supper that will dazzle your family and friends but don't have the time to sweat over the stove, this dish is a fantastic option. The honey and soy glaze gives the fish a sweet and savoury coating while also adding some excitement to your wilted greens side dish.

HONEY, 1 TABLESPOON

• 3 TEASPOONS SOY SAUCE WITH LOW SODIUM

• A 114-POUND SKINLESS SALMON FILLET CUT INTO 4 PARTS

• SALT AND PEPPER, FRESHLY GROUND

• CANOLA OIL (1 TABLESPOON)

- 1 SEEDED AND THINLY SLICED RED BELL PEPPER

- 1 TABLESPOON FRESH GINGER, CRUMBLED

- PACKED SPINACH (12 CUPS)

Preheat the broiler. Combine honey and 1 teaspoon soy sauce in a small mixing dish. Place aside.

2. Use aluminium foil to line a broiler-safe baking dish. Season the salmon with salt and pepper before serving. Broil the fish for 5 minutes on a baking dish. Broil for another 2 to 5 minutes, until salmon is cooked through and flaky.

3. Heat oil in a large nonstick skillet over medium-high heat while the salmon broils. Cook for 3 to 4 minutes, or until bell pepper has softened. Stir in the ginger until everything is fully blended. Season spinach with salt and cook for 2 minutes, or until wilted. Add the remaining 2 teaspoons soy sauce and mix well. Serve with the salmon.

Chapter Twenty-eight

Wraps with smoked salmon and cream cheese, spinach, and artichokes

SERVES 4

- EACH SERVING CONTAINS 397 CALORIES

- TOTAL TIME TO PREPARE: 12 MINUTES

This dish is a heart-healthy power recipe, with fiber-rich whole-wheat wraps, omega-3-rich smoked salmon, and vitamin-packed spinach. These wraps provide 43 grammes of protein per serving and will keep you satisfied.

- REDUCED-FAT CREAM CHEESE (12 CUP)

- 2 TABLESPOONS FRESH DILL, CRUMBLED

- 2 TABLESPOONS FRESH CHIVES, CRUMBLED

- FRESHLY GROUND PEPPER (14 TEASPOON)

- 4 WRAPS OF WHOLE GRAIN

SMOKED SALMON, 8 OUNCES

CAPERS (2 TABLESPOONS)

SUNFLOWER SEEDS, 3 TABLESPOONS

• 1 CUP ARTICHOKE HEARTS, SLICED

• 2 CUP BABY SPINACH, PACKED

Combine cream cheese, dill, chives, and pepper in a large mixing bowl. Distribute the mixture evenly among the wraps. Layer one-fourth of the salmon, capers, sunflower seeds, artichoke hearts, and spinach in each wrap to finish making the sandwiches. Roll each wrap securely and cut in half.

Chapter Twenty-nine

Chicken Breasts, Pan-Fried

SERVES 4

• EACH SERVING CONTAINS 92 CALORIES

• TOTAL TIME TO PREPARE: 13 MINUTES

These chicken breasts are easy to prepare in quantity and store in the refrigerator for use in everything from omelettes to salads throughout the week. Season arugula with salt, pepper, and a squeeze of lemon for a tasty, low-calorie companion to this entrée. Pounding the chicken breasts according to the recipe will assist them to cook more quickly and evenly.

• FOUR BONELESS, SKINLESS CHICKEN BREASTS, HALVED, 4 OUNCES

• SALT (12 TEASPOON)

• FRESHLY GROUND PEPPER (12 TEASPOON)

• OLIVE OIL (2 TEASPOONS)

1. Sandwich the chicken breasts between two heavy-duty plastic wrap sheets. Pound the chicken breasts with a meat mallet or rolling pin until they are about 12 inch thick. Season with salt and pepper on both sides.

2. Heat oil in a large nonstick skillet over medium-high heat. Cook for 3 minutes on each side, or until light golden and cooked through.

Chapter Thirty

Lemon and Garlic Breaded Chicken Thighs

SERVES 4

• EACH SERVING CONTAINS 172 CALORIES

• TOTAL TIME TO PREPARE: 26 MINUTES

Although chicken breasts are the leanest cut of the bird, they aren't the only component you can utilise to make healthful recipes. Go to the dark side if you want your chicken dish to have more flavour. Thighs have a few more calories than chicken breasts, but they're juicier, more tender, and even cheaper.

• 4 SKINNED CHICKEN THIGHS

• 1 TABLESPOON FLOUR (ALL-PURPOSE)

• SALT (14 TEASPOON)

• FRESHLY GROUND PEPPER (14 TEASPOON)

• 1 WHITE EGG, LIGHTLY BEATEN

1 TABLESPOON WATER

• 12 CUP BREAD CRUMBS WITH ITALIAN SAUCE

• OLIVE OIL (2 TEASPOONS)

• 12 CUP LOW-SODIUM FAT-FREE CHICKEN BROTH

• ½ CUP WINE IN WHITE

• FRESH LEMON JUICE (2 TABLESPOONS)

2 FINELY MINCED GARLIC CLOVES

• 2 TABLESPOONS FRESH PARSLEY, CRUMBLED

• 1 TABLESPOON DRAINED CAPERS

1. Combine chicken, flour, salt, and pepper in a heavy-duty sealable plastic bag. Shake the bag to evenly coat the chicken. Whisk together egg white and water in a shallow basin. Bread crumbs should be placed in a separate shallow basin.

2. Take 1 chicken thigh from the bag and dip it in the egg white mixture before dredging it in bread crumbs. Place aside. Rep with the remaining chicken.

3. Heat oil in a large nonstick skillet over medium heat. Cook the chicken for 3 minutes on each side, bone side up, or until browned. Bring the broth, wine, lemon juice, and garlic to a boil in the pan with the chicken. Reduce the heat to low

and cover for 8 minutes. Cook, uncovered, for 5 minutes, until chicken is cooked through, adding parsley and capers as needed. Serve right away.

Chapter Thirty-one

Chicken Breasts Stuffed with Goat Cheese and Sun-Dried Tomatoes

SERVES 4

• EACH SERVING CONTAINS 296 CALORIES

• TOTAL TIME TO PREPARE: 55 MINUTES

You don't have to eliminate cheese from your diet just because you're watching your calories. Goat cheese is a tangy and flavorful alternative to cow cheeses like cheddar, and it's also lower in fat, calories, and cholesterol.

• 1 CUP WATER IS BOILING

• 13 CUP SUNDRIED TOMATOES WITHOUT THE OIL

• OLIVE OIL (2 TEASPOONS)

• DIVIDE 12 CUP CHOPPED SHALLOTS

• SUGAR (112) TEASPOONS

3 MINCED GARLIC CLOVES

• DIVIDEd BALSAMIC VINEGAR (212 TABLESPOONS)

• ½ CUP (ABOUT 2 OUNCES) GOAT CHEESE CRUMBLED

• 2 TABLESPOONS FRESH BASIL, CRUMBLED

• SALT (34 TEASPOON)

• FOUR CHICKEN BREAST HALVES, 6 OUNCES

• FRESHLY GROUND PEPPER, 18 TEASPOON

• FAT-FREE, LOW-SODIUM CHICKEN BROTH (34 CUP)

• DRIED THYME, 14 TEASPOON

CORNSTARCH, 2 TEASPOONS

• WATER (2 TEASPOONS)

1. Combine boiling water and tomatoes in a small bowl. Allow to sit for 30 minutes, or until soft. Drain and chop finely.

2. Heat 1 teaspoon oil in a large nonstick skillet over medium heat. 13 cup shallots, sugar, and garlic, sauté until golden brown, 4 minutes Combine the shallot mixture and 112 tablespoons vinegar in a large mixing basin. Toss in the chopped tomatoes, cheese, basil, and 14 tsp salt and mix well.

3. Cut a horizontal incision into the thickest section of each chicken breast piece with a paring knife or steak knife. 2

teaspoons tomato mixture, stuffed into each slit Sprinkle salt and pepper over the chicken.

4. Heat the remaining 1 teaspoon oil in a large nonstick skillet over medium-high heat. Cook for 6 minutes on each side, or until chicken is thoroughly cooked. Take the chicken off the heat. Bring broth, thyme, remaining shallots, and vinegar to a boil in the same pan. Combine cornstarch and water in a small mixing dish. Bring the cornstarch mixture to a boil in the pan. Cook, whisking continually, for 1 minute, or until sauce thickens slightly. Serve the sauce over the chicken.

4 SERVINGS • 202 CALORIES PER SERVING
PROSCIUTTO-WRAPPED CHICKEN

• TOTAL TIME TO PREPARE: 19 MINUTES

While dried herbs can easily be replaced for fresh herbs, missing out on the flavour of sage in this meal would be a pity. As one of the key ingredients, the earthy herb definitely shines. Also, as indicated, stick to low-sodium chicken broth—the prosciutto adds plenty of salt to the dish.

• FOUR CHICKEN CUTLETS, 4 OUNCES

• SALT, 18 TEASPOON

12 SAGE LEAVES, FRESH

• 2 OUNCES PROSCIUTTO, THINLY SLICED INTO 8 THIN STRIPS

• DIVIDE 2 TABLESPOONS OLIVE OIL

• FAT-FREE, LOW-SODIUM CHICKEN BROTH (13 CUP)

• ¼ CUP LEMON JUICE, FRESH

WEDGES WITH 12 TEASPOON CORNSTARCH (OPTIONAL)

1. Salt and pepper the chicken. On one side of each cutlet, arrange three sage leaves; secure the sage by wrapping each cutlet in two slices of prosciutto.

2. Heat 1 tablespoon oil in a large skillet over medium heat. Place the chicken in the pan and cook for 2 minutes on each side. Keep the chicken heated in the skillet.

3. Whisk together the broth, lemon juice, and cornstarch in a small mixing basin until smooth. Add the broth mixture and the remaining oil to the same skillet where you cooked the chicken. Bring to a boil while constantly whisking. Cook for another minute, whisking frequently, until the sauce has thickened somewhat. Pour the sauce over the cooked chicken. With lemon slices on the side (if using).

Chapter Thirty-two

Jambalaya with sausage and chicken

SERVES 4

• EACH SERVING CONTAINS 341 CALORIES

• TOTAL TIME TO PREPARE: 45 MINUTES

This Creole-inspired recipe will have a lot of flavour right away, so make it the day before you want to consume it. The dish will truly sing after the flavours have had chance to blend.

• CANOLA OIL, 2 TEASPOONS

• 6 OUNCES REDUCED-FAT SMOKED CHICKEN SAUSAGE, CUT INTO 14-INCH SLICES LENGTHWISE

• ½ CUP ONION, CRUMBLED

12 CUP CELERY, CRUMBLED

12 CUP GREEN BELL PEPPER, CRUMBLED

2 MINCED GARLIC CLOVES

• 1 CUP LONG-GRAIN WHITE RICE, UNCOOKED

1 CUP OF WATER

• 14 TEASPOON RED PEPPER, GROUND

• SALT, 18 TEASPOON

6 SPRIGS FRESH THYME

• ONE FAT-FREE, LOW-SODIUM CHICKEN BROTH 14.5 OUNCE CAN

• ONE 14.5-OUNCE CAN UNDRAINED TOMATOES WITHOUT SALT

• 1 CUP CHICKEN BREAST SHREDDED ROTISSERIE

Heat oil in a Dutch oven or large pot over medium heat. Brown sausage in a skillet for 1 minute. Cook for 6 minutes, until onion, celery, bell pepper, and garlic are softened. Bring to a boil the rice, water, red pepper, salt, thyme, and chicken broth. Reduce the heat to low, cover, and cook for 20 minutes, or until the rice is tender. Cook for 3 minutes, or until tomatoes and chicken are heated through. Before serving, remove the thyme sprigs.

Chapter Thirty-three

Sandwich with Sliced Apples and Open-Faced Turkey and Havarti

SERVES 4

• EACH SERVING CONTAINS 427 CALORIES

• TOTAL TIME TO PREPARE: 10 MINUTES

This sandwich is a terrific crowd-pleaser because to the sweet apples, acidic Havarti, and spicy arugula. If you don't like mustard, leave it out of this recipe; the sandwich will still be wonderful without it.

• 4 BREAD SLICES

• 4 TEASPOONS MAYONNAISE (LOW-FAT)

• DIJON MUSTARD, 4 TEASPOONS

• 1 CUP ARUGULA

• FOUR RED ONION SLICES, 18 INCHES THICK

- 12 OUNCES DELI TURKEY, THINLY SLICED

- 2 APPLES, CORED AND CUT INTO EIGHT 14-INCH-THICK SLICES CROSSWISE

- ½ CUP (2 OUNCES) HAVARTI CHEESE, GRATED

- PEPPER, FRESHLY GROUND

Preheat the broiler.

2. Spread 1 teaspoon mayonnaise and 1 teaspoon mustard on each slice of bread to make sandwiches. 14 cup arugula, 1 onion slice, 3 ounces turkey, 4 apple pieces, and 2 tablespoons cheese should be layered on each.

3. Transfer the sandwiches to a baking sheet with a spatula. Broil for 4 minutes, or until bubbling cheese. Remove from the fire and season with a pinch of black pepper. Serve right away.

Chapter Thirty-four

Turkey Burgers with Teriyaki Onions Sauté

SERVES 4

- EACH SERVING CONTAINS 278 CALORIES

- TOTAL TIME TO PREPARE: 35 MINUTES

Replace ground beef with ground turkey to lighten up a basic burger. This recipe incorporates sweet and savoury onions, which are a wonderful complement to the feast for traditionalists who believe turkey lacks flavour.

- GROUND TURKEY BREAST (1 POUND)

- GARLIC POWDER (2 TEASPOONS)

- CAJUN SEASONING (1 TEASPOON)

- FRESHLY GROUND PEPPER (14 TEASPOON)

- LIGHT TERIYAKI SAUCE (3 TABLESPOONS)

• 1 WATER TABLESPOON

• SPRAY FOR COOKING

1 LARGE ONION, CUT IN 14-INCHES SLICES

• OLIVE OIL (1 TEASPOON)

• 4 BUNS DE HAMBURGER

• EIGHT 14-INCH TOMATO SLICES

• 4 LEAVES OF LETTUCE

1. Combine ground turkey, garlic powder, Cajun seasoning, and pepper in a large mixing basin. Form the mixture into four patties.

2. Combine teriyaki sauce and water in a small bowl.

3. Spray a big nonstick skillet with cooking spray and heat on medium. Cook the onions in a covered skillet for 10 minutes. 1 tablespoon teriyaki sauce (diluted) Set aside the onions from the pan.

4. Heat the oil in the same skillet over medium heat. Cook for 5 minutes on each side of the turkey patties. Fill the pan with the remaining 3 tablespoons of diluted teriyaki sauce. Flip patties with a spatula and cook for 3 minutes, or until lightly browned.

5. To assemble the burgers, place one patty on the bottom bread of each bottom bun. 14 cup sautéed onion, 2 tomato

slices, and 1 lettuce leaf on top of each. Finish with the bun's top.

Chapter Thirty-five

Tenderloin de Porc Rosemary-Garlic

SERVES 4

- EACH SERVING CONTAINS 147 CALORIES

- TOTAL TIME TO PREPARE: 30 MINUTES

There are lots of additional lean protein options if you've had your fill of chicken breasts. Pork tenderloin is a reasonably inexpensive option, and when cooked properly, "the other white flesh" is soft and moist. As this recipe demonstrates, only a few ingredients are required to infuse the pork with flavour.

- 2 TABLESPOONS FRESH ROSEMARY, FINELY CRUMBLED

- 4 MINCED GARLIC CLOVES

- 1 POUND TRIMMED PORK TENDERLOIN

- SALT (12 TEASPOON)

- FRESHLY GROUND PEPPER (14 TEASPOON)

• SPRAY FOR COOKING

Preheat the oven to 475 degrees Fahrenheit.

2. Combine the rosemary and garlic in a small bowl. Cut multiple slits into the pork loin using a paring knife or steak knife. Half of the garlic mixture should be stuffed into the incisions. Wrap the pork loin with the leftover garlic mixture. Salt & pepper to taste. Using nonstick cooking spray, coat a jelly roll pan or baking sheet. Insert an oven-safe meat thermometer into the thickest portion of the tenderloin and place it on the pan.

3. Bake tenderloin for 20 minutes, or until slightly pink. The internal temperature of the beef should be around 160°F. Before slicing the tenderloin, remove it from the oven and let it rest for 5 minutes.

Chapter Thirty-six

Mustard-Caper Sauce Pork Chops

SERVES 4

• EACH SERVING CONTAINS 491 CALORIES

• TOTAL TIME TO PREPARE: 30 MINUTES

This recipe demonstrates how a tasty sauce may be produced fast, without the use of butter or flour, and with only a few ingredients. The salty capers, acidic mustard, and fragrant rosemary combine to provide a flavorful and pleasing pork accompaniment. To liven up a plain side dish, sprinkle some additional sauce over cooked vegetables.

• OLIVE OIL (1 TABLESPOON)

• 4 BONE-IN PORK LOIN CHOPS (TOTAL WEIGHT: 312 POUNDS), 1 INCH THICKNESS

• SALT (12 TEASPOON)

- FRESHLY GROUND PEPPER (12 TEASPOON)

- 2 CUPS CHICKEN BROTH WITH LOW SODIUM

- 112 TABLESPOONS WHOLE-GRAIN MAYONNAISE

- 3 TABLESPOONS RINSED CAPERS

- 14 TEASPOON FRESH ROSEMARY, CRUMBLED

1. Heat oil in a large frying pan over medium heat. Season both sides of the pork with salt and pepper. Cook for 10 minutes on each side, or until the centre is just pink. Place the chops in a serving plate.

2. Pour broth into the same pan and bring to a boil over high heat. Combine the mustard, capers, and rosemary in a bowl. Reduce heat to low and cook sauce for 4 minutes, or until it has reduced by half. Serve the pork with the sauce.

Chapter Thirty-seven

Meatballs with Peppers of Three Colors

SERVES 4

- EACH SERVING CONTAINS 263 CALORIES

- TOTAL TIME TO PREPARE: 30 MINUTES

Ground round steak, which is around 85 percent lean, is used in this dish. Although it is not as lean as sirloin (which is roughly 90% lean), the slight variation in fat content will result in juicier meatballs. To save time, you can instead use store-bought bread crumbs in place of the whole-wheat bread slice.

- 1 CUP GREEN BELL PEPPER, THINLY SLICED

- 1 CUP RED BELL PEPPER, THINLY SLICED

- 1 CUP YELLOW BELL PEPPER, THINLY SLICED

- 113 CUP + 14 CUP WATER

- 10.5-OUNCE BEEF BROTH CAN

• 1 BAY LEAF

• 1 WHOLE-WHEAT BREAD SLICE

• GROUND ROUND STEAK, 1 POUND

• 1 TABLESPOON ONION, FINELY CRUMBLED

• DRIED OREGANO (12 TEASPOON)

• SALT (12 TEASPOON)

• FRESHLY GROUND PEPPER (12 TEASPOON)

• 1 WHITE EGG

1 CRUSHED GARLIC CLOVE

• OLIVE OIL (2 TEASPOONS)

• 2 TABLESPOONS FLOUR (ALL-PURPOSE)

• 13 CUP FRESH BASIL, FINELY CRUMBLED (OR 112 TEASPOONS DRIED)

• 2 TEASPOONS VINEGAR (WHITE)

1. Combine the bell peppers, 113 cup water, broth, and bay leaf in a large pot. Bring to a boil, then decrease heat to low. Cook for 20 minutes on low.

2. Pulse the bread in a food processor to make approximately 12 cup coarse crumbs while the peppers simmer. Combine bread crumbs, meat, onion, oregano, salt, pepper, egg white,

and garlic in a large mixing bowl until well combined. Make 1-inch meatballs out of the beef mixture; the recipe should make 36.

3. Heat oil in a large nonstick skillet over medium-high heat. Cook meatballs for about 10 minutes, or until all sides are browned.

4. Combine flour and remaining water in a small bowl. Stir the flour mixture into the peppers in the saucepan. Cook, stirring regularly, for 3 minutes after adding meatballs to pan. Remove the bay leaf and combine with the basil and vinegar. Serve right away.

Sliders of beef with pita and hummus

EACH SERVING CONTAINS 488 CALORIES

• TOTAL TIME TO PREPARE: 15 MINUTES

This dish combines small ground beef patties with a healthy portion of hummus for a unique take on the slider craze. Serve alongside a simple bed of romaine seasoned with red wine vinegar and a little drizzle of olive oil, with a few feta crumbles on top, to make this dish even more Mediterranean.

• LEAN GROUND BEEF (1 POUND)

• DRIED OREGANO, 112 TEASPOONS

• SALT AND PEPPER, FRESHLY GROUND

- OLIVE OIL (2 TABLESPOONS)

- 4 PITAS WITHOUT A POCKET

- 34 CUP HUMMUS FROM THE STORE

14 SLICES SMALL RED ONION

- 2 TABLESPOONS PARSLEY FLAT-LEAF

- WEDGES OF LEMON

1. Form 16 half-inch-thick tiny patties from the beef. Add oregano, salt, and pepper to taste.

2. Heat 1 tablespoon oil in a large nonstick skillet over medium heat. Cook for 2 minutes on each side, or until done to your liking.

3. To build the pitas, divide the hummus evenly among them. Top each pita with four burgers, onions, and parsley. Serve with a lemon wedge and a sprinkle of oil on each pita.

Chapter Thirty-eight

Salad of Beef Stir-Fried with Avocado and Black Beans

SERVES 4

• EACH SERVING CONTAINS 436 CALORIES

• TOTAL TIME TO PREPARE: 10 MINUTES

Stir-frying your meat and vegetables is a simple and healthy method to make a one-pot meal. Cotija cheese is a dry, salty, sharp Mexican cheese that can be substituted with Parmesan or Asiago in this recipe.

• BEEF TENDERLOIN, 12 OUNCES, SLICED INTO THIN STRIPS

• DIVIDE 14 CUP FRESH LIME JUICE

• 12 TEASPOON CHILI POWDER PLUS 1 TABLESPOON

• VEGETABLE OIL (1 TABLESPOON)

• THINLY SLICED MEDIUM SWEET ONION

- 1 SEEDED, DERIBBED, AND THINLY SLICED RED BELL PEPPER

- 1 SEEDED, DERIBBED, AND THINLY SLICED POBLANO PEPPER

- SALT (12 TEASPOON)

- FRESHLY GROUND PEPPER (12 TEASPOON)

- RINSED AND DRAINED ONE 15-OUNCE CAN BLACK BEANS

- 1 DICED AVOCADO

- 14 CUP COTIJA CHEESE, CRUMBLED

- 14 CUP FRESH CILANTRO CHOPPED

1. Combine meat, 2 tablespoons lime juice, and 1 tablespoon chilli powder in a large mixing basin; put aside.

2. Heat oil in a large nonstick skillet over medium heat. 5 minutes, tossing periodically, onion, bell pepper, and poblano Cook for 3 minutes after adding the beef. Salt & pepper to taste.

3. Combine beans, avocado, cheese, cilantro, the remaining lime juice, and the remaining 12 teaspoon chilli powder in a separate mixing dish. Salad should be served alongside the steak and vegetables.

Chapter Thirty-nine

Balsamic Tomato Sauce on Sliced Flank Steak

SERVES 4

• EACH SERVING CONTAINS 246 CALORIES

• TOTAL TIME TO PREPARE: 20 MINUTES

While some kinds of meat can wreak havoc on a calorie-restricted diet, flank steak is a lean, low-calorie option for a healthy diet. This recipe is great all year, but it shines in the summer when basil and tomatoes are at their peak.

• OLIVE OIL (1 TABLESPOON)

• TRIMMED 1 POUND FLANK STEAK

• SALT (12 TEASPOON)

• FRESHLY GROUND PEPPER (12 TEASPOON)

3 MINCED GARLIC CLOVES

- 1 MINCED SHALLOT

- ¼ CUP VINEGAR BALSAMIC

- 2 CUPS QUARTERED CHERRY TOMATOES

13 CUP FRESH BASIL, CHOPPED, DIVIDED

- DIVIDE 13 CUP THINLY SLICED GREEN ONIONS

1. Heat the oil in a large skillet over medium heat. Season the meat with salt and pepper before serving. Cook for 5 minutes on each side, or until desired doneness is reached. Remove the steak from the grill and place it on a chopping board. Allow for 5 minutes of resting time before slicing thinly against the grain.

2. In the meantime, sauté the garlic and shallot in the same skillet over medium heat. Cook until gently browned, about 1 to 2 minutes. Pour in the vinegar and heat for 1 to 2 minutes, or until the liquid is nearly gone. Add the tomatoes, 14 cup basil, and 14 cup green onions and stir to combine. Cook, stirring periodically, for 2 minutes. Pour the tomato mixture over the meat once it has softened. Serve immediately with the remaining basil and onions.

Chapter Forty

Restaurants

The 5:2 Diet is extremely adaptable. Fast days can be scheduled around any time you need to eat out. However, plans sometimes change, and you may find yourself dining out on a fast day. So having a few menu item selection strategies is beneficial. Consider these options:

• Salads without croutons, cheese, or avocado, with the dressing on the side

• Steamed, poached, roasted, or grilled dishes—avoid pan-fried, battered, breaded, au gratin, deep fried, creamy, or crispy menu items.

• No sauces, toppings, or marinades on the menu

• Skinless chicken breast, pork tenderloin, or seafood

• White-egg dishes

- Sandwiches made with lean meats and vegetables

- Meals from the children's menu

- Salsa, mustard, or flavoured vinegars seasoned meals

- Side dishes, or request that half of your meal be wrapped before being served.

- Foods cooked in olive oil rather than butter or shortening

You may replace lower-calorie options for some of your favourite restaurant dishes no matter what meal you're having. Because most restaurants are aware of dietary restrictions, inform your waitress that you require low-calorie and low-fat advice. The majority of establishments will gladly satisfy your wishes. Keep in mind that different restaurants utilise different recipes for their menu items, so the substitution chart below can be used as a guide. A excellent suggestion is to place your order first so that your choices are not influenced by what others order. People regularly duplicate orders in restaurants because they want to fit in socially, according to studies. The following are some good low-calorie restaurant alternatives:

CPSIA information can be obtained
at www.ICGtesting.com
Printed in the USA
BVHW061829180722
642397BV00012BB/336